Spanking Contract & Agreement

This book and its contents are for entertainment purposes only. This is not a legally binding contract. Warning - Even if a Spanking and/or BDSM contract is not considered legally binding in your country/locality, attempts may be made to include parts of it in law enforcement or other legal proceedings, should their involvement ever occur for some reason. "Consent" could be a defense to assault in many places (though not necessarily effective.) A legal argument might be attempted stating that by signing the contract you are agreeing to everything in it. Also, in areas of the world where some or all BDSM activities are illegal, contracts of any sort can be used to prosecute those involved.

This book is sold and/or distributed with the understanding that the publisher and author is not engaged in rendering legal or other professional services. **The writer, publisher and distributors of this publication expressly disclaim all liability for the use of this publication and/or the interpretation by anybody of information contained in this publication.** The author, publisher and distributors of this publication hereby disclaim any and all liability for any loss or damage caused by errors or omissions resulted from negligence, accident, or any other causes. This book and its subject matter are for entertainment purposes only. In this publication there may be inadvertent inaccuracies including technical inaccuracies, typographical inaccuracies and other possible inaccuracies. If legal advice or other expert assistance is required, the services of a competent professional person in a consultation capacity should be sought. Products, services and websites' content vary with time. Please verify any published information.

Spanking Contract & Agreement

Copyright © 2013 by Phil G.

ISBN-13: 978-1492792208
ISBN-10: 1492792209

Erotic BDSM Books - Your Erotic BDSM Book Publisher
EroticBDSMbooks.com

I0426041

This publication comes with two free bonus books.
Your books are presented in this order:

Other BDSM Books by Phil G. Include:

*BDSM Master/slave Contract

*Mistress/slave BDSM Contract

*The Absolutely Essential Book of BDSM and S&M Rules
*Things To Do During 3 Hours of Sex; A Step-by-step Guide
*Playtime At The Dom Den; A Step-by-step Guide
*The Absolutely Essential Guide to Great BDSM and S&M Sex
*The Absolutely Essential Dominant/submissive Playtime Experience
*The Absolutely Essential BDSM Sexual Experience
*The Ultimate Collection of S&M and BDSM Rules For Female Submissives and Slaves
*Master and submissive or slave BDSM Contract
*The Funniest BDSM Personal Ads
*Have Awesome BDSM Sex
*Spanking Dictionary
*BDSM Rules
*Bed Arrest, the Punishment for BDSM Enthusiasts

Spanking Contract and Agreement

Table of Contents

Introduction

A *Spanking Contract and Agreement* is a document that presumably outlines the terms of the relationship in regard to spanking and many or all directly related subjects. The contract is considered an important part of the commitment that a couple shares and makes as part of that lifestyle. Both the Spanker and spankee sign the agreement indicating their commitment to one another and the terms of the agreement. Both Spanker and spankee should feel free to change and amend this contract in a mutually acceptable manner.

A standard employment contract (which this isn't) optimally adapted for this endeavor might have a better chance of standing up in court. It is of course presumed that legal issues will not arise from your relationship (as typically they don't.)

The spankee should not enter into this contract unless he/she is sure (from experience) that she enjoys being spanked as well as feels secure with the other signing party.

This agreement must be entered voluntarily, but cannot be broken except under the conditions stated in the contract.

Trust, care, mutual consent, safe sex practices, and general safety are absolute priorities. No matter what, it's suggested that you incorporate at least the following into your playtime and lifestyle:

- Don't tie things around someone's neck, and no breath play, period!
- Create a "Safe word" for the submissive to say when (or if) things get too scary.
- Always be careful and take necessary safety precautions when engaging in BDSM activity. Keep proper medical facilities handy.
- Always insure that a bound person has adequate circulation. If the person tied up has to go to the bathroom or has physical problems, that person must be immediately released from bondage.
- Ask about medical issues before playing and adjust your playing activities according to any medical issues.
- Never leave anyone bound and alone.
- Understand what a gagged person sounds like in sexual ecstasy versus in pain.
- Do not play while under the influence of drugs or alcohol.
- Always check that your handcuffs and/or lock keys work before playing. If you have to go to the locksmith to get the handcuffs off, it's going to be embarrassing.
- When removing someone from bondage, allow them to move their own limbs.
- If pregnant or ill, check with your doctor before engaging in BDSM related activity.
- Always play within your own skill base and comfort level.

This collection is only a guide. You should add, subtract and adapt rules as desired. There is ample room for that. If you live with others, such as children, it's likely many rules will at least need to be adapted.

Make changes by (1) crossing out the rule and writing into the contract its substitute in the blank space at the end of this section or (2) just crossing out the wording and writing in the new word or words above or below it. (Using white-out and writing over the white-out is an alternative also.)

1. Rules Governing Time In and Time Out of this Contract

Definition of Time In - spankee: "Time In" refers to the period of time the spankee is subject to terms and conditions of this contract. *Time In* is to be considered in effect at all times when the spankee is in the Spanker's presence or communicating with him in any way.

Definition of Time In - "Time In" refers to the period of time the Spanker and/or spankee are subject to terms and conditions of this contract.

Definition of Time Out: "Time Out" refers to specific periods of time when the spankee and/or Spanker is **not** subject to the terms and conditions of this contract. The following rules apply to this *"Time Out"* period:

The Spanker may call a "Time Out" any time he/she wishes. (This "time out" can be for a specific period of time or an open-ended period of time.)

The spankee may request a "Time Out" for a specific period of time only. The spankee must state her/his reasons and the time period for the request and await the Spanker's permission for the Time Out. Should her Spanker not grant the Time Out, her only option is to end her relationship with her Spanker.

2. Definition of a Spanking

The act of hitting (slapping) the buttocks for punishment and/or pleasure. Corporal punishment is to given to sting the flesh effectively without truly harming the spankee in any way. To do this correctly the buttock must be scrutinized closely and be well maintained.

3. Contract Start Date & Duration

This contract will be in force indefinitely, or if not, from:

_____ (*the start date*)

to the following day (*optional – include the time*):

_____ (*the end date*).

Witness Printed Name and Signature (*optional*):

_____

If the contract is noted as temporary, at the end of the stated duration of this contract, both parties will decide whether to renew the contract, and/or change the contract, and/or let the contract elapse completely.

Duration - This contract will be in force until one or both parties' consider it null and void.

This *Spanking Contract and Agreement* remains valid on all points for the length of the contract unless otherwise amended.

I. Specifically For the Spankee

(Make changes by (1) crossing out the rule and writing into the contract its substitute in the blank space at the end of this section or (2) just crossing out the wording and writing in the new word or words above or below it. (Using white-out and writing over the white-out is an alternative also.)

4. Spankee Signature *(Spanker's signature is in another section further in the document)*

I, _____

(Spankee should write and print name here)

(Circle one or more of the following) - Wife of, slave of, submissive of, girlfriend of and/or boyfriend of:

_____

(Print name of Spanker)

Do hereby acknowledge that I have read this *Spanking Agreement and Contract* completely and approve and accept all the doctrines it advocates. From this date on it is my wish to have my spanking implemented, enforced and regulated by the doctrines in this *Spanking Agreement and Contract*.

Therefore I give to _____
(print Spanker's name), the full right and permission to spank me whenever he/she feels such discipline/spankings would prove helpful and is be in accordance with this *Spanking Agreement and Contract*.

I have entered into this *Spanking Agreement and Contract* willingly and with sound mind. I understand that I can expect to be spanked without fail if I fail to up-hold commitments I make in this contract.

*I and my partner's (the Spanker's) spanking related activities are private and confidential. Neither Spanker nor spankee is allowed to divulge **any** information that implies or states that spanking occurs, without both parties expressed permission and on each occasion.*

Both parties acknowledge that they are aware of the possible consequences of what is stated in this agreement and accept those consequences. **(This contract has nothing to do with minors and was not written to be incorporated by parents spanking their minor kids.)**

5. Rule of Consent

No spanking may given before a third party without the FREE CONSENT and WILLING permission of both parties before it's occurrence. It will always remain a secret that such discipline is ever even administered (spanking and domination) without the FREE CONSENT and WILLING permission of both the Spanker and spankee. This spanking Agreement and Contract is meant to be a private and intimate agreement that is part of the (preferably) love and (definitely) compassion for your partner.

6. Personal Acknowledgements of the Spankee

A. I acknowledge that I am a spankophile (somebody who gains satisfaction, sexual and/or otherwise in some form or another from spanking) and that a primary reason that my buttock even exists is to be spanked. At least at times I will want to be spanked in a manner that makes my bottom look and feels well spanked. This means my buttocks can be made red or pink and have some marks on them.

B. I have been spanked enough times as an adult and with a hard enough intensity and duration to know I want to be spanked as much, and at least at times, as hard as this agreement states.

C. I hereby give my Spanker the right to spank me for any other reason that *is or is not* specifically stated in this Spanking Agreement and Contract. This includes when he/she just wishes to spank me for no other reason than it is his/her desire at the moment.

D. When I am to be spanked I promise to fully cooperate with my Spanker. I will get ready for the spanking promptly when told to do so and I will present myself to him/her in the manner demanded by him/her (and/or as described in this contract) with no ill feelings towards the Spanker. During and after the spanking I will also hold no ill feelings toward my Spanker if he/she sticks to the terms of this contract.

E. I agree to be spanked by open palm, flogger, leather slapper, strap, paddle, cane, switch, carpet duster, hairbrush, bathroom brush, wooden spoon, leather strap, ruler, belt, cat of nine tails and slipper. Any spanking implements that have not previously been discussed in this contract must have the expressed okay for use by both parties.

F. My Spanker has the right to make my butt pink/red whenever he/she spanks me. I accept that my butt, or at least part of it, could become pink and/or red during and after any of my spankings. If I'm being spanked hard, switched or caned, bruises and/or welts could appear on my buttocks. These are to be avoided if possible (though this becomes difficult if I bruise easily.) No blood or blisters are allowed from being spanked or otherwise beaten. If periodically something of this nature does occur it can be forgiven by the spankee. (How easily the spankee bruises also depends on how fragile the spankee's body is and how used to being spanked the spankee is. In time most asses toughen up from being spanked often and this could become less of a concern.)

Marks – (*Spanking Marks*) – A good spanking with more than moderate intensity (depending on how sensitive the spankee's bottom is) can leave the bottom a lovely shade of red. It also can also leave light contusions and more significant bruises. These bruises (aka "marks") could remain for days or longer or they can be gone in hours. A spankophile is proud of these marks hence the phrase "wears her (his) marks with pride".

Spankings given to leave marks must have the spankee's permission to occur.

G. The duration and intensity of a spanking, and what my Spanker uses on my bottom, is always the choice of my Spanker. I may however discuss something that concerns me at anytime regarding this, as well as make pertinent requests.

H. Should I feel that my Spanker is too sadistic and/or unstable I will end my relationship with that person or otherwise protect myself from that person.

I. I promise to take steps to keep my spanking relationship active and lively. Among other things, I will (along with my Spanker) provide new spanking implements and/or spanking furniture as well as new ways to be tied up, and tied down, for my spankings.

J. I will do my best to keep my bottom as spank-friendly as possible. Working out the buttock muscles can make my butt look firmer.

K. I will take great pride in being about to take a good, hard spanking. It may take me some time for my bottom to be able to take a good hard spanking but it is something my Spanker has the right to expect from me and I want to be able to take.

L. I will keep my ass clean and smelling fresh prior to my spankings (unless perhaps the spanking occurs spontaneously).

M. I will quickly put myself into any spanking position that my Spanker wants me to be in, including over his lap, over a chair, on the bed and in the spanking wheelbarrow position.

N. By default, I will call my male Spanker "Sir" at least just prior to, during and just after the spanking process. If my Spanker is female, by default I will call her "Maam" at least just prior to, during and just after the spanking process. If my Spanker wants me to call him/her something else, I will call him/her that instead.

O. I understand that if I am a submissive or slave, there will likely be additional rules for me to obey that are not in this contract. Perhaps I should also get at my bookstore one of the following contracts: "**BDSM Master/slave Contract**" or "**Mistress/slave BDSM Contract**".

P. I will promptly take the position that my Spanker orders me to, or my default position is to wait for my spanking by kneeling in front of him/her while he/she is sitting on something (like a chair or couch.) When kneeling in front of him/her, if requested, I will make sure to have my breasts exposed for his/her pleasure. I will also have my hands behind my back (or neck if the Spanker prefers) so as to be out of the way.

Q. I will always be on time to the appointed time and location for my spanking. If not I should expect to be punished for that.

R. I will not purposely be a brat to get a spanking.

S. My bottom can be made wet to possibly increase the pain level of the spanking.

T. I always will be at the appointed location and at the appointed time to receive my spanking from my spankee, with the exception of emergencies.

U. I will obediently and quickly present my naked bottom whenever my Spanker wants (assuming the privacy requirements of this contract is adhered to) for him/her to check to see how my previously well spanked bottom is doing and/or for him/her to spank. This does not promise the Spanker full access to my bottom for sexual purposes.

V. I will never refuse or delay the disciplinary process by fibbing, such as by saying I have a headache, too much female period pain or feel significantly unwell when that's not the case.

W. I will not block my Spanker's spanks (and/or hands) or try to get away from a position my Spanker has ordered me to be in unless there is an emergency or I am in harm's way. Should my Spanker ever spank my hand because it was blocking a blow, I will be spanked much harder and longer and perhaps have my hands bound in front of me, or punished in an additional way. I may also get a breast spanking as further punishment. I will also have the humiliation of knowing I was so disrespectful.

X. If my Spanker wants me to get, or otherwise move spanking implements and/or punishment/spanking related objects, possibly in preparation for a spanking, that is what I will promptly do.

Y. Most spanks (slaps to the buttocks) are to land on my buttocks only, though some spanks may sometimes land on my upper legs.

Z. If my health is suffering, such as I have a bad enough headache, I can insist that I don't get spanked and my Spanker must not spank me. I am never allowed to exaggerate this problem or worse yet make up an ailment to get out of a spanking.

AA. If I <u>want</u> to be spanked, my Spanker is *required* to spank me ASAP. However I need to tell my Spanker that I want to be spanked and not try to convey that desire in a less direct manner.

7. Privacy

A. All spankings that I receive must be done in a private setting where only people I'm comfortable with are in and/or outside the room I'm being spanked in. Only people I'm comfortable with can hear any aspect of my spanking, including scolding, the impact of hand and/or spanking implement on my person.

B. My spanking partner's spanking related activities are private and confidential. Neither party is allowed to divulge any information that implies or states that it occurs without his/her expressed permission on each occasion.

8. Who Else May Spank Me

I hereby allow my Spanker at anytime to decide who else can spank me, as long as I am (initial which is/are pertinent, or by default, without your explicit permission, your Spanker can only let someone spank you if you're fully clothed):

1) Fully dressed _____ (initial if you agree)
2) Fully dressed and/or when I only have panties on _____ (initial if you agree)
3) Fully dressed and/or when I only have panties on and/or when my buttocks are naked but I am clothed otherwise _____ (initial if you agree)

4) Fully dressed and/or when I only have panties on and/or when my buttocks are naked but I am clothed and/or when I am fully naked _____ (initial if you agree).

9. Intensity and Duration of My Spankings

A. I hereby allow my Spanker to decide how hard my spankings will be.

B. I hereby allow my Spanker to decide for what length my spankings will be.

C. I hereby allow my Spanker to decide how often I will be spanked.

D. If my Spanker tells me that I am to get a certain number of spankings in a set time period (such as a week) it will be my responsibility to make sure to remind my Spanker to give them to me. Should my Spanker fail to give those particular spankings to me then it is the Spanker's right to reschedule them.

10. Sexual Aspects of Spanking

A. Spanking my buttocks as part of foreplay and during sex is always allowed.

B. I agree to let my Spanker play with my body, including my pussy, clitoris and breasts at anytime as part of spanking me. This includes the use of sex toys. Finger vibrators, when put on a finger of the hand not spanking me, can be put against my clitoris while I'm being spanked for a (presumably) great sensation.

C. Thinking about the spanking that awaits me will turn me on sexually.

D. My pussy (If the spankee is female) must be wet within 90 seconds into any spanking. No spanking (other than quick playful spanks) will ever end until my pussy is wet.

E. *Sexually Oriented Spankings* - Sexually Oriented Spankings are spankings that are specifically given to make the spankee orgasm or at least get as much sexual pleasure as possible.

Intercourse may occur later but more specifically her orgasm is done by fingers (including her own if the Spanker allows it) and/or sex toy(s). Typically the spanking ends when the spankee is done cumming.

I can always ask for a *Sexually Oriented Spanking* but should not expect them on a regular basis. My Spanker is not under any obligation to give me such spankings but should if he/she is a good Spanker.

F. It is my Spanker's decision as to if I can masturbate before, during and immediately after the spanking.
G. I am always allowed to look at pornography except for specific cases that may offend my Spanker.

H. Assuming we are in a place with privacy, after any spanking by my Spanker I will service him/her sexually if my Spanker wants it. What type of sexual activity we do will be determined by my Spanker.

It is my opinion that if someone is being kind enough to give me the discipline and spankings I so badly need, it is my job to make sure he/she is sexually satisfied from the experience.

11. *Orgasming From Being Spanked*

If my Spanker wishes he/she will train me to orgasm from being spanked. Most submissive spankees can be trained to orgasm from being spanked and as a respectful submissive spankee I will learn to orgasm for my Spanker while being spanked. Within 3 minutes into the spanking, I will naturally start to orgasm without clitoral or vaginal stimulation. (If I am the Spanker's submissive or slave, I will ask for permission to cum first of course). My Master/Mistress can instead order me to start my orgasm during the spanking at anytime. As a submissive or slave I will always need permission to stop my orgasm.

For training me to cum from being spanked, my Spanker will likely start by using a vibrator on me during the spanking. My Spanker acknowledges that I may need up to 10 training sessions with a vibrator in this manner. After then, should I disrespect my Spanker by not cumming when ordered to while being spanked, (assuming I was given permission to cum,) then I will be separately punished.

B. During my spanking, a foremost thought in my mind will be giving sexual pleasure to my Spanker. I will however always need permission to play with his/her cock, pussy or breasts before, during and after my spanking.

12. *Spanking the Spankee's Breasts.*

My Spanker may spank my breasts in a manner consistent with this contract. Spanking of my breasts however is always done in a consensual manner so that I can have it stopped, altered or not allowed at anytime unless it is noted otherwise here:

13. Mood Correction & Maintenance Spankings

MAINTENANCE SPANKINGS – (*Preventative Maintenance Spankings*) – These are spankings administered on a regular basis to keep the spankee on the straight and narrow. Punishment spankings are administered in addition to these.

MOOD CORRECTION SPANKING – When a spanking(s) is administer to alter the mood of the spankee. Perhaps the spankee is in a bad mood. A mood correction spanking is then administered in an attempt to alter his/her perspective/attitude. More than one mood correction spanking can be given and given between relatively short time intervals.

When my Spanker and I are together, if I feel that I am getting into a bad mood, I'm to ask for a "*Mood Correction Spanking*" from my Spanker. This rule is repeated every five minutes until the mood changes. Should my Spanker think I need yet another mood correction spanking and I fail to ask for another spanking within 5 minutes, I will receive a caning or a breast spanking instead. I promise to request spankings, whether they are maintenance spankings or not, when I feel I need them.

14. Domestic Discipline

This is not a specific *Domestic Discipline Agreement/Contract* per se but with this contract the spankee agrees to accept spankings at the discretion of the Domestic Discipline Spanker per the stipulations laid out in this agreement. All other aspects of this contract also pertain to the Domestic Discipline relationship.

15. Punishment and Punishment Spankings.

A. If my spanking has been a punishment spanking and if my Spanker requires it from me, I will obediently tell him/her what I have learned from that discipline. I will respect my Spanker's advice in regard to how to resolve my unacceptable behavior. If I think of them, I will provide us with strategies as to how I won't repeat what got me disciplined in the first place.

If at any time my Spanker wants to discuss any aspects related to my discipline, including that/those specific situations that got me disciplined, I have no choice but to openly and honestly discuss it with my Spanker, even if it could get me punished further. This discussion must be in private and according to the confidentiality agreed upon in this contract.

B. If I know I have acted in an unacceptable manner in the opinion of my Spanker I will be anxious to be spanked/punished for it. This means I must tell my Spanker about it if he/she didn't already know.

C. Once a punishment spanking has been announced it is not up for debate, any whining or complaining of any sort will add extra to the punishment. I may request that the spanking be put off but it is the Spanker's decision if it is to be administered now or later.

D. Any crying I do while being spanked for punishment (if I need to cry at all) will simply be a turn on for my Spanker and will not affect the length or to an extent, intensity of my punishment. If I cry while being punished it likely means I'm learning my lesson. The exception is when I'm experiencing physical pain from other correctable sources. For instances if my hands are tied and my shoulder is in a painful position, I should always feel free to tell my Spanker about that and my Spanker is obligated to immediately take me out of that situation that is causing me that pain. Reasonable pain from being spanked however is not something that can be negotiated (assuming this point has been agreed upon by both parties.) If I do not like the kind of pain my Spanker ever gives me directly from being spanked, I need to find another Spanker or leave the spanking lifestyle. My Spanker however should rarely be putting me in that position.

E. It is my Spanker's decision whether to combine punishment spankings with other types of punishment such as corner time, bed arrest, etc. I will not resist these other punishments that I've been sentenced to assuming those meet any related criteria laid out in this contract.

16. Spanking as a Reward. I can always ask that my reward (assuming I'm due a reward from my Spanker) be a *Sexually Oriented Spanking* or at least just a spanking.

17. Spanking Clothing Related

A. I am not allowed to wear panties in the home if my Spanker is present. Exceptions are when I could be embarrassed from it such as when company is there or expected. My Spanker can check to see if I'm wearing panties or not at anytime (that coincides with the terms of this agreement.)

B. If we are in private, my Spanker can always require me to change into attire he/she would prefer. (This includes me being naked.) I have no choice in the matter and will promptly comply. This includes putting my hair in the appropriate hairdo such as pigtails if I'm dressed up as a schoolgirl.

C. I will wear spank-friendly underwear when my Spanker wants me to (except in situations where that underwear could be exposed to others such as in a fitness club locker room). The definition of spank-friendly underwear is what my Spankers decide it is.

D. I will wear dresses or skirts when and if my Spanker wants that.

E. I will get at least one schoolgirl outfit (if I don't have one) if my Spanker wants me to.

F. While we are in private, I will not wear a bra if my Spanker does not want me too.

18. Lying Across the Spanker's Lap to Relax

My Spanker may require I lay across his/her lap while he/she is watching TV or reading, etc. This way my bottom is there for him/her to spank and/or play with at his/her leisure. (As has already been noted, I am required to remove my clothing when my Spanker wishes me to so I could be without clothing lying over my Spanker's lap.) The book he's/she's reading (if a book is being read) would rest on my bottom. I will comply with this order promptly. I may initiate it myself by asking permission to do it.

19. Resistance Associated With the Spanking

A. During the spanking I will always be respectful. This includes never attempting to block blows from the spanking to my bottom. If I kick my feet it will not be enough to block the spanks on my bottom. If my Spanker orders me to lessen or stop any of my physical reactions to being spanked, I will.

Should I fail to stop impeding the blows to my buttocks or moving too much or otherwise making it more difficult for my Spanker to physically spank me, I should expect my naked breasts to also be spanked and/or much more punishment.

B. I will not make what my Spanker considers to be too much noise as a reaction to being spanked.

20. Additional Things That Can Get Me Spanked

A. If my Spanker wants it (or agrees to it) whenever I and/or my Spanker and I come back from being in the public, I am to ask for a *"returning from the public spanking."*

This spanking is to be administered no matter how many other spankings the spankee has recently gotten. Also, it is the spankee's responsibility to remind the Spanker for these.

B. Whenever I am to leave the house (apartment or where ever) for more than just quickly going to the car, or something quick of that nature, whether I'm also leaving with my Spanker or not, I will ask my Spanker for a *"going out in the public spanking."* This is over and above any other spankings I may have recently received or am going to receive soon.

C. When alone with my Spanker, unless he/she has told me to do otherwise, I am to ask every hour, at the beginning of the hour, to be spanked for "my hourly spanking," no matter whether I've been spanked recently or not. My Spanker may not want to spank me but I'm required to ask roughly on the start of each hour anyway.

21. *Preparing for the Spanking*

A. I will take the position that my Spanker orders me to, or my default position is to kneel in front of him/her while he/she is sitting. When kneeling in front of him/her I will make sure to have my breasts exposed for his/her pleasure, if my Spanker wants that. I will also have my hands behind my back (or neck if the Spanker prefers) so as to be out of the way and make playing with me easier. My legs will be spread moderately making access to my pussy easier.

B. If I am to be spanked, preparing to be spanked, or being scolded, out of respect I will not allow my eyes to look above my Spanker's midsection.

C. If my Spanker wants me to I will count out each (or as many as he/she wishes) spanks as/after they're administered.

D. It is my Spanker's decision as to whether I will undress myself or if he/she will remove any or all of my clothing (or if someone else will remove my clothing, assuming that is allowed in this agreement.)

E. If the spankee wants a spanking to be delayed or called off, her only recourse is to beg for that as well as be as sexy as possible while begging.

F. At any time my Spanker may tie my hands together and/or tie me to the bed/furniture to better immobilize me so as to make the spanking easier and more fun, for the Spanker at least.

22. *During the Spanking*

A. During, before and/or after the spanking my Spanker may at anytime order me to "spread 'em" which means I am to spread my legs so he/she can better spank my inner butt as well as have better access to my pussy and anus.

B. *Clenching* (*Clenching Cheeks*) is allowed by the spankee – *Definition*: This is when the spankee tightens his/her buttocks muscles together forcefully. This might be done in an attempt to dull the sting of the spanking.

C. Just prior to, during and immediately after all of my spankings, my Spanker may play with and enjoy my pussy, breasts and anus as he/she wishes (assuming the proper sanitation proceedings are adhered to as well as any other terms of this contract.)

D. I will apologize to my Spanker during any punishment spanking process, assuming I feel that way and/or my Spanker orders me too.

23. Post Spanking

A. After and during a spanking my Spanker has the right to rake my sore and/or red bottom with his fingernails, or use a related instrument to do that instead. Extreme care must be taken to not break the skin. Should that occur by accident the wound must be cleaned with antiseptic and the priority is that it be allowed to heal, thus making spanking that specific area of the buttocks off limits until the healing process is complete.

B. After a punishment spanking, my Spanker has the right to rub my bottom with sandpaper or have me sit naked on sandpaper. Extreme care must be taken to not break the skin. Should that occur by accident the wound must be cleaned with antiseptic and the priority is that it be allowed to heal, thus making spanking that specific area of the buttocks off limits until the healing process is complete.

C. I will apologize to my Spanker during and/or as part of the post spanking process, assuming I feel that way or my Spanker orders me too.

D. At least periodically, after a spanking, I will thank my Spanker for having taken the trouble of spanking me.

E. It is my responsibility to put away, keep clean and keep organized our spanking implements and sex toys. This includes BDSM equipment.

F. Rubbing my spanked bottom is always allowed unless my Spanker specifically states I can't for that particular spanking.

24. Silent Spanking (Capsaicin Cream Use)

(Results vary from individual to individual) – *My Spanker has the right to do this to me*: Applying a *very small* amount of this cream onto the naked buttocks is an alternative to spanking (thus is called "*Silent Spanking*"). It seeps into the bottom and often is painful. A surprisingly small amount is needed. Make sure to quickly wash your hands after applying it or you will be in pain too. (Better yet use something else to apply it with.)

Rub the *capsaicin cream* in well. It might take some time to make its impact well noticed. Spankers I suggest you first experiment by rubbing a tiny bit into your spankee's butt. Only drops of it would be necessary to first test his/her resistance to it. Olive oil or vegetable oil can help dissipate the pain. This cream may look innocent but the stuff is *evil*! (Tiger Balm is another possible punishment cream.) Do not put any of this on or in the anus or vagina!

If the spankee is going out in public, he/she can refuse *capsaicin cream* (or the like) being put on her (though it's great fun to watch her squirm in public this way.)

25. Exercise Spanking

If the spankee needs motivation to exercise and/or exercise harder, spanking can be of use. The spankee can be spanked whenever exercise goals are not reached and/or can get the more desirable reward of a pleasurable spanking when the goals are met. My Spanker has the right to give me exercise spankings as he/she sees fit.

26. Spanking Outdoors

The spankee is allowed to be spanked outdoors whenever the Spanker wishes, assuming privacy is assured and all other related aspects of this contract are adhered to.

27. Motivational Spankings

The spankee agrees to take *Motivational Spankings* as her Spanker thinks she/he needs them. This type of spanking scenario can help the spankee reach his/her goals. Perhaps the goal is good grades in college, or weight loss, or quitting smoking. Motivational spankings can work (but like anything in life is not guaranteed to work.)

A. Before the spankee embarks on their endeavor he/she can be given the first motivational spanking, which is a serious spanking that really show him/her that it's better to stick with the program. Remember, his/her subconscious mind needs to be motivated also and a really good spanking might do just that.

B. Should the spankee fail to reach previously established goals, he/she should be very soundly spanked and otherwise punished. Other punishments can include corner time, not being allowed to wear cloths (when in private,) Bed Arrest, orgasm denial and other forms of humiliation can also be incorporated. Perhaps you'd also like to invite all your BDSM/kinky friends over to give him/her a spanking.

28. Pussy Spanking

If the spankee allows it, the vagina can be lightly spanked for stimulation and/or punishment.

29. Schoolgirl Spanking

The naughty (adult) schoolgirl discipline fantasy is one of the most popular spanking fantasies. She is dressed in the pleated skirt and white dress shirt (perhaps also with a tie) and is constantly getting in trouble so she is constantly spanked! All female spanking enthusiasts (spankees) should have a schoolgirl outfit!

The Spanker can require this of the spankee if he/she wants.

30. Maid Service Spanking

(Definition - Spankee is dressed up as a maid and does house cleaning, typically with a strict Spanker making sure she/he does a really good job and if she doesn't....hmmmmmmmm.)

If the Spanker wants this the Spankee will do it as often as the Spanker wants.

31. *Miscellaneous Additional Rules*

A. This spanking contract does not allow for more than some embarrassment and shame. If emphasizing embarrassment and shame, an additional/alternative agreement will be needed, unless it is acceptable with the spankee. Of course there is at least some embarrassment and shame involved in punishment spankings but when most of the punishment is to embarrass and/or shame the spankee, another agreement regarding that likely is necessary.

B. The Spanker is at full liberty to add alternative/additional punishment activities to the spanking scene (that are also allowed according to the terms of this contract.) These include:

1) Making the spankee stand in a corner after and/or in between spankings
2) Spanking her breasts and/or pussy (if that is allowed by this contract)
3) Bed Arrest
4) Not being allowed to wear cloths (if privacy is assured)
5) Not being allowed to wear underwear for a set period of time, even when in a public setting
6) Not being allowed to wear a bra
7) Writing a sentence over and over again
8) Make the spankee do some extra cleaning somewhere.

C. *Dropseat Pajamas* - If my Spanker wants me to get and wear these, at least from time to time, I will get them and wear them, at least from time to time - *Definition*: These pajamas open at the buttocks for excreting waste and spanking.

D. *Enema Spankings* is allowed only when the spankee allows it. *Definition*: combining enemas with spankings. The spankee is given a spanking then an enema is administered. The spankee releases the water and immediately gets another spanking.

E. *Heating Pad Use on the Spanked Butt* – This is allowed. *Definition* – (1) After a good spanking, if additional punishment is warranted, laying the heated pad over the well spanked buttocks might be the answer. (2) The spankee could place his/her butt on the heating pad before the spanking possibly making it more tender. (3) For some, sitting on the heating pad can feel like punishment.

Additional Rules & Notes

II. Specifically For the Spanker and Spankee

Make changes by (1) crossing out the rule and writing into the contract its substitute in the blank space at the end of this section or (2) just crossing out the wording and writing in the new word or words above or below it. (Using white-out and writing over the white-out is an alternative also.

1. If a punishment spanking is given, both parties (the Spanker and spankee) agree to immediately resume good relations right after the spanking is over. (Perhaps relations were always good and thus there would be no need for this rule.) To hold a grudge or to continue a quarrel or misunderstanding after a spanking has been administered, is not allowed for either the Spanker and/or spankee.

2. Both parties promise to cooperate with each other fully and faithfully in carrying out this agreement.

3. Taking pictures or videos of the Spanker and/or spankee, or any part of either party, is only allowed when the party whose picture is being taken gives expressed permission for each picture, reproduction and/or instance of video taking. Thus for every individual picture taken of the Spanker and/or spankee, she/he needs to give permission. The face or any other identifying marks are not allowed in any picture without the express permission of the person who's picture is being taken. Thus permission must be given for every picture and every time a picture is taken. This also holds true for drawings or other reproductions of the spankee.

4. No picture or other type of reproduction of either parties may be publically or privately circulated without the expressed permission of ball parties.

5. Care should be administered when one or more parties are angry with each other. It's best to wait until both parties are calmer and then carry out the punishment.

6. If the use of a safe word is integrated into this relationship, the Spanker agrees to immediately stop spanking the spankee when he/she says the safe word.

7. If the person who is normally the Spanker, reverses the roles and allows him or herself to get spanked for some reason (perhaps because he/she feels the need to be punished for something,) then the person administering the spanking (who is normally the spankee) will adhere to all the rules the normal Spanker is required to obey according to this contract.

8. The two of you will find your favorite places in the abode for the spankings to take place. Maybe it's over the desk, on the bed, over a wooden spanking horse, over the Spanker's lap, over the back of a chair, etc.

9. If the Spanker wants, a journal will be kept of how often the spankee is spanked, the intensity level of the spanking and why the spankee was spanked. It is the Spanker's decision as to who keeps the journal but both the Spanker and spankee can read it at anytime.

10. Punishment Agreements - A punishment agreement for the specific punishment to be given for various infractions that are committed by the spankee, can be established ahead of time. (It is however the right of the Spanker to add additional punishment to those predefined punishments as well as vary the intensity of any spanking.)

Should the spankee commit any of the offenses defined in the punishment agreement the spankee gets the punishment that's been agreed upon. (Again, it is the right for the Spanker to add to the punishment or decrease its severity should he/she wish it. In most cases however that is to be frowned upon.)

This punishment agreement you create is valid for as long as it is part of this Spanking Contract and this Spanking Contract is valid.

Offenses that the spankee can get a pre-established type of spankings for (and/or other types of punishment) include:

*Inattentiveness
*Being rude (unnecessarily)
*Not doing established housework or doing it properly
*Being late for any commitment
*Not wearing the proper/or otherwise ordered to wear attire
*Lying
*Being a brat
*Insubordination at home, work or at another place (unnecessarily)
*Stealing
*Not sticking to a diet or weight loss program
*Breaking something
*Being bitchy
*Not putting herself in the required spanking position fast enough
*Failure in some manner as a lover however small. (In the mind of the Spanker.)
*Not looking good and/or as sexy as could reasonably be expected for her Spanker
*Doing something poorly
*Cheating
*Less than acceptable hygiene
*Not being as sexy or seductive enough for her Spanker
*Failure to swallow her Spanker's cum
*Pouting
*Whining

*Being drunk (if not allowed)
*Being late
*Getting a traffic ticket
*Ogling another person in a manner that offenses her Spanker
*Over use of the telephone or being online too much
*Add additional infractions and the pre-established punishment here:

III. Specifically For the Spanker

Make changes by (1) crossing out the rule and writing into the contract its substitute in the blank space at the end of this section or (2) just crossing out the wording and writing in the new word or words above or below it. (Using white-out and writing over the white-out is an alternative also.

32. Spanker Signature

I, _____

(circle which of the following is pertinent) - husband of, BDSM owner of, dominant of, girlfriend of

and/or boyfriend of the spankee _____
do hereby acknowledge that I have read this *Spanking Agreement and Contract* and approve and accept all the doctrines it advocates.

I have entered into *this Spanking Agreement and Contract* willingly and with sound mind. I promise to uphold the commitments I made in this contract.

33. Miscellaneous Spanker Rules

In addition to the previously stated, I the Spanker agree as to the following:

A. To take care not to cut the spankee's skin, raise welts (that don't fade in a timely manner) or otherwise bruise or injure his/her body.

B. That any punishment spanking should continue long enough and be of the appropriate intensity to be effective and provide a beneficial lesson to my spankee partner. I want to give her/him responsible discipline, not mindless abuse.

C. For my spankee's own good, I promise to discipline her/him without fail and as quickly as possible whenever she/he violates any of the terms of this agreement.

D. I promise to help take steps to keep my spanking relationship active and lively. I will (along with my spankee) provide new spanking implements as well as new ways to tie up, and tie down, my spankee.

E. I am allowed to look at pornography except for specific cases that offends the spankee.

F. I will be at the appointed location and at the appointed time to administer the spanking to my spankee with the exception of emergencies.

G. Hand spankings might convey more intimacy but it remains my right (the Spanker) to choose what to spank the Spanker with.

H. It is my decision as the Spanker if I want to pick a regular day and/or night that the previous week's punishment spanking, or spankings will be given to the spankee. For instance, if the spankee misbehaved on Tuesday, perhaps it is preferred that her spanking be put off and given on the upcoming Friday night. (This gives the spankee something to think about in anticipation.) That way if my spankee also misbehaved between Wednesday and Friday night, she would get double the punishment that Friday night!

I. I have the right to spank my spankee at anytime as long as it is within the confines of this agreement. Perhaps some issues require both an immediate spanking as well as a spanking during the weekly spanking catch-up night just mentioned in "H".

J. If the spankee requests a spanking and notes the intensity level she/he wants, I as the Spanker AM REQUIRED to give it to her/him ASAP.

K. It is only the Spanker that can delay or decide against giving a spanking, assuming the situation is within the confines of this agreement.

L. It is the Spanker who decides how much of the spanking is going to be given either on the spankee's bare bottom or alternatively on her partially or fully clothed bottom.

M. It is the Spanker who has the final word on what spanking implements are going to be used on the spankee.

N. The Spanker will feel free to use *soothing cream* (i.e. cold cream which is a cream applied to a well spanked bottom to limit the sensation of pain) on the spankee's butt after the spankee has been well spanked. It is the Spanker's choice as to whether to use it or not.

Additional Rules and Notes

The End

By Phil G.

Book #2 – The Spanking Dictionary

The Spanking Dictionary

Caution is always advised in anything related to spanking, discipline and punishment. Always stay within legal boundaries.

Spanking pronouns, (which include names of spanking websites, spanking actors/actresses, spanking parties and spanking media) are NOT included in this dictionary due to space limitations. **Spanking of minors is not discussed in this book nor advocated.**

ADULT SPANKING - Spanking taking place among and between people who are of legal age.

ADULT SPANKING SCENARIOS - Spanking activities that take place among adults. These are often thought up and set up ahead of time.

AMATEUR SPANKING – (1) Unless a person is spanking, or receiving spankings for money or other material gain (such as Spanking Therapists and professional FemDoms do,) then this category includes most in the adult spanking world. (2) While not all agree on this angle of the definition, it has been used to imply a Spanker or spankee who is not proficient in the spanking arts.

ANAL EXAM – The dominant spends a lot of time inspecting, testing and ultimately using the spankee's anus for his/her pleasure.

ANGER MANAGEMENT THERAPY SPANKING - Spanking can be used as a kind of therapy to help manage anger. There are two different approaches.

(1) The angered/stressed person is the *spankee* and gets spanked for a length and an intensity that allows the anger/stress to be released. Multiple spankings may be needed.

(2) The angered/stressed person is the *Spanker* and spanks for a length and an intensity that allows the anger/stress to be released. Multiple spankings may be needed.

ANNIVERSARY SPANKING - Like birthday spankings this involves a tradition where as part of the festivities one or multiple participants spank and/or get spanked. It may include a special sexual scenario also. Spankophiles might want to get creative and have these anniversaries occur on other anniversaries such as when the couple met, became engaged and/or had their first date.

AVERAGE SPANKING (An) – Your basic everyday spanking, the usual. (Yawn.)

BARE BOTTOM SPANKINGS – Applying the spanking directly to the uncovered buttocks. There are advantages to this versus spanking the covered buttocks:

1) *Better access*; the Spanker may wish to use the spankee's bottom for other types of stimulation including anal and vaginal stimulation. The Spanker may want to rub the naked bottom sensually at various times, etc.

2) *Humiliation*; the spankee must expose him/herself.

3) *Intensity*; clothing can lessen the impact of the blows and thus lessen the spanking's sensation and/or ability to provide punishment.

4) *Safety*; All parties can see how the buttocks is fairing from the blows. Perhaps the intensity needs to be lessened; you might not know if the buttocks are covered.

BARE BOTTOM BEATING – See *Bare Bottom Spankings*.

BATHBRUSH – A long handled brush used for washing one's self during bathing. It can be an effective spanking tool.

BEDROOM TIME – Being banished to the bedroom after, and/or as part of a punishment spanking. Often this bad girl will get spanked more than once while serving bedroom time.

BED ARREST – A type of BDSM punishment. See "*Bed Arrest, the Punishment for BDSM Enthusiasts*".

BEDTIME SPANKING – (1) Spankings irregularly administered as foreplay to sex prior to going to sleep for the night. (2) Spankings which are administered nightly (or irregularly) when the spankee and/or Spanker goes to bed, whether there is to be sexual activity or not.

A number of spankees claim a bedtime spanking helps make them sleepy.

BEHAVIOR MODIFICATION SPANKING – Spanking(s) administered to change unwanted behavior. Repeated and hard spankings may well be necessary to make this work.

BELT – It holds a man's pants up and is a nasty spanking implement. You're in for it now young lady!

BIRCHING – Birching is to spank using a tied together collection of thin tree switches. A nice touch is to have the spankee go out and pick the tree switches herself and tie them together securely for future use or use as soon as it is made.

BIRTHDAY SPANKING - A "traditional" birthday spanking is given on the birthday of the spankee. The formula is to administer one swat for each year of age, plus one additional swat "to grow on, one to live on, one to be happy on, to get married on, etc." The last swat can be the hardest as it's for any bad behavior that he/she did last year.

Spankee beware! Many will say that each birthday party attendee gets to give the same number of spanks, which can make for hundreds of spanks!

The spankee might pick and choose who gets to do the spanking and birthday spankings are typically done clothed as it's often done at children's parties.
Birthday spankings are usually done by hand but if it involves consenting adults spanking that often won't be the case.

Dominants may want to incorporate "practice birthday spankings" with their submissives as another excuse to spank.

Birthday spankings can be given belatedly but typically are for only the spankee's previous birthday (not all his/her birthdays.)

Blindfolding the adult spankee might be a nice touch.

A "*Reverse Birthday Spanking*" is when the person having the birthday gets to give the spankings instead!

BOARD OF CORRECTION – Slang name for a paddle.

BOTTOMS UP – While more known as a saying for drinking everything from a glass (container) so the bottom of the container is pointing up (thus sending all the liquid into your mouth,) this also means presenting a bottom for a spanking.

BOTTOM RAKING - Sliding your fingernails over and across the spanked or unspanked ass. This should not be done hard enough to puncture the skin or even take any layers of skin off. This should also only be done over the fleshy part of the buttocks and not near the anus or sexual organs.

BROKE THE PADDLE ON MY BUTT – This saying can be put in different ways. It's a source of pride for the spankee that when someone spanked his/her butt using a paddle, the paddle broke upon hitting his/her butt.

BRUTAL SPANKING – See *Severe Spanking*.

CAPSAICIN CREAM – (Results vary from individual to individual.) - Applying a *very small* amount of this cream onto the naked buttocks is an alternative to spanking (thus is called "*Silent Spanking*"). It seeps into the bottom and often is painful. A surprisingly small amount is needed. Make sure to quickly wash your hands after applying it or you will be in pain too. (Better yet use something else to apply it with.)

Rub the *capsaicin cream* in well. It might take some time to make its impact well noticed. Spankers I suggest you first experiment by rubbing a tiny bit into your spankee's butt. Only drops of it would be necessary to first test his/her resistance to it. Olive oil or vegetable oil can help dissipate the pain. This cream may look innocent but the stuff is *evil*! (Tiger Balm is another possible punishment cream.) Do not put any of this on or in the anus or vagina!

CANING – This is when a cane is applied with force to the buttocks of the spankee. The cane can hurt more than many other spanking implements due to its smaller surface area so caution is advised. Also see *Switching*.

CARPET BEATER – A long handled housekeeping tool used to beat dust off of hanging rugs and to spank worthy bottoms.

CHARITY SPANKING - Charity Spanking is when people are spanked in exchange for others sponsoring them and giving money to one or more charities for each good spank they take. Also see *Professional Spanking*.

CLENCHING – (Clenching Cheeks) – This is when the spankee tightens his/her buttocks muscles together forcefully. This might be done in an attempt to dull the sting of the spanking.

COMING BACK IN FROM THE PUBLIC SPANKINGS – After the spankee returns to a private secluded setting, after having been in the public (and that includes having been to work or having been shopping), she gets a spanking as a natural course of events. This is over and above any other spankings she's getting for any other reason. This is associated with but the opposite of *Going Out in the Public Spanking*.

CONFESSIONAL {THERAPY} SPANKING - (1) A religiously related spanking scene where the Spanker plays an authoritative person of religious faith who spanks the spankee in an effort to get him/her to be more religiously righteous or pay for his/her sins. This may be more popular in Domestic Discipline households. (This happened for real a lot more in centuries past than most hear about.)

(2) The spankee perhaps was raised in a strict religious environment and needs that type of strict (and perhaps regular) guidance to stay on the straight and narrow. A good spanking once or twice a week for just this could be a pleasant addition to your relationship. This obviously has similarities to the confessional of Catholics and doing penance.

(3) In an attempt to get the spankee to confess to something, he/she is spanked. Once he/she confesses then punishment would be administered, which would be another type of spanking such as *Punishment Spanking*.

CONFIDENTIAL SPANKING – The spanking partners agree to keep their spanking relationship and other spanking related activities secret, except to whom they both agree on. It is essential to follow this rule.

CONSENSUAL SPANKING – Informed and agreed-upon spanking that takes place between and among consenting adults.

CORPORAL PUNISHMENT – This is physical punishment inflicted on the human body. This includes spanking but can also include the death penalty.

CROP – A slapping instrument originally meant to urge horses to move. It can be a wonderful spanking implement.

CRUEL TO BE KIND – A saying that is loosely associated with the potentially beneficial impact of adult spanking.

DETENTION ROOM – This is where many naughty schoolgirls go in spanking films and fantasies. This is the location of much discipline, primarily spanking.

DISCIPLINARIAN – Someone with authority that dispenses discipline, often by giving spankings.

DISCIPLINE - It incorporates punishment to correct disobedience of the rules and/or other unacceptable behavior.

DIZZY SPANKING - For this kind of spanking, the spankee is spun around on foot or in a chair that can spin around, until he/she is dizzy. The spankee is then spanked. This is for healthy spankees only and it's essential to take care for safety.

DOMESTIC DISCIPLINE – (*Christian Domestic Discipline, Spanking for Jesus, Loving Domestic Discipline*) – This typically is discipline relegated for couples, and often is administered in Christian dominated households. Rules are instituted and penalties for disobedience are administered. The male tends to be the dominate person (*Head of Household* [HOH]).

DOMINATION SPANKING – The spanking often includes additional aspects of domination such as oral commands, punishment and physical restraint.

DROPSEAT PAJAMAS – These pajamas open at the buttocks for excreting waste and spanking.

DUEL SPANKING - (*Tandem Spanking*) - This is a *Spanking Contest* between spanking couples. The spanking is done simultaneous or one at a time. See *Spanking Contest*.

ENDURANCE SPANKING - This can be done to determine the spanking length and intensity limits of a spankee. (Of course limits change with time.) How much can the spankee take, how many swats, how hard can the swats be, how long can the spanking go on? Are there certain spanking implements that the spankee doesn't do as well with?

Spanking models often go through this unless they have good references.

ENEMA SPANKINGS – Combining enemas with spankings. The spankee is given a spanking then an enema is administered. The spankee releases the water and immediately gets another spanking.

EROTIC SPANKING - Erotic Spanking are spanking activities and techniques that are executed expressly to enhance sexual pleasure. Admittedly spanking (even the thought of spanking) likely enhances a spankopile's pleasure but with *Erotic Spanking* it's taken a step further. For instance the couple can alternate spankings with the use of a variety of sexual toys and/or manual sexual stimulation.

The spankee can be securely tied down so she/he is immobile and can be enjoyed in other ways after and in-between spankings.

EXERCISE SPANKING – If the spankee needs motivation to exercise and/or exercise harder, spanking can be of use. The spankee can be spanked whenever exercise goals are not reached and/or can get the more desirable reward of a pleasurable spanking when the goals are met.

EXHIBITION SPANKING – This is when spanking models, professional or amateur, provide the public with a spanking related show. The spankee(s) could be clothed or exposed. Also see *Public Spanking*.

EXORCISM SPANKING – ("Exorcism Beating") - This occurred historically in various places and times in both western and eastern orthodox Christianity, as well as in other religions. This also occurred as part of the inquisitions. In most cases however, the spankee was lucky if their main punishment was only being spanked (beaten.)

Over the centuries some clergy members, particularly those that still were allowed to have sex, set up chambers where women were spanked, sometimes on a sizable wooden cross, for their purported transgressions. It might have been just one spanking or a semi-regular occurrence.

The spankee's buttocks may or may not be exposed for the beating and onlookers may or may not be allowed to watch, or even aid in the beatings.

F/f SPANKING – Female spanking female.

F/m SPANKING - Female spanking male.

FIFTY SHADES OF GREY - A groundbreaking, famous 2011 erotic romance novel by British author E. L. James. Its erotic scenes include BDSM activities such as bondage, discipline, dominance/submission, sadism and masochism.

FIRM HAND – The Spanker has a strong and likely big hand that can deliver impressively hard spanks.

FLOGGING – A flogger is a variation of the cat-of-nine-tails whip. It's typically made of suede or real leather and has many individual elastic strands attached to the handle.

GOING OUT IN THE PUBLIC SPANKING – Before the spankee goes out into the public (and that includes going to work or shopping), she gets a spanking as a natural course of events. This is over and above any other spankings she's getting for any other reason. This is associated with *Coming Back in from the Public Spankings*.

GOOD OLD FASHION SPANKING – These are the standard spankings we grew up with. *Silent Spankings* and many if not all spankings when the Spanker is tied down to spanking furniture, likely are not in this category. This term denotes a hard or harder than normal spanking.

GROUP SPANKING – When a multiplicity of people conjugate for the expressed purposes of engaging in one or more kinds of spanking and spanking related endeavors.

HALLOWEEN SPANKING – Spanking on Halloween while people are in costume. Ideally the spankee(s) should not know who's doing the spanking. Another version has it that the spankee(s) are the ones that people can't tell the identity of.

HAIRBRUSH – (Hated Hairbrush) – The household hairbrush makes a very effective and surprisingly intense spanking tool. Mmmmmm!

HAND SPANKING – Directly applying the spanking blows to those naughty butt cheeks with your hand(s).

HANDPRINT – On a well spanked red ass, if the Spanker lands a single hard spank, a white handprint on the otherwise red ass cheek might appear for a short time.

HARD SPANKINGS – A true spankophile should be able to take a hard spanking, at least from time to time. Hard spankings might only be relegated for punishment. Technically a hard spanking should not have the intensity of a severe spanking. Depending however on the pain threshold level of the spankee, a hard spanking could make a spankee cry.

Hard spankings however may evolve into your norm. You may find it best to tie down the spankee for a hard spanking.

The Spanker can make demands of the spankee during a hard spanking, demands that need to be promised to be met before the spanking can stop. Perhaps by using a vibrator in her anus she would be required to cum before the spanking could stop.

Unless the spankee has very developed resistance, his/her bottom should be red and perhaps marked from a hard spanking.

If the spankee is female it's suggested that no hard spanking ever ends unless her pussy is wet just from the spanking and she's promising to be a very good girl!

HEATING PAD – (1) After a good spanking, if additional punishment is warranted, laying the heated pad over the well spanked buttocks might be the answer. (2) The spankee could place his/her butt on the heating pad before the spanking possibly making it more tender. (3) For some sitting on the heating pad can feel like punishment.

HOLIDAY SPANKING – Spankings in some cases can really add to the holiday cheer! (Of course there's always *Spanking Santa* in his red outfit!)

HOT SPANKING – Spanking that are more sexually stimulating than most.

HOUSE PADDLE – A paddle that is kept readily available as a courtesy for guests to use. (It can be another spanking implement instead and named accordingly).

HUMILIATION THERAPY SPANKING – Sometimes a person needs more humility, one way to give him or her more humility is to combine domination with long, hard spankings. Or just a long hard spanking could do the trick. Spanking Therapists and FemDoms can specialize in this.

ICE SPANKING – There are variations to this spanking technique. If you're interested you and your partner should experiment and find the way that works best for you.

The spankee will need to have her buttocks fully exposed. The Spanker can do any of the following, or combine them:

a) First rub ice on/across her naked buttocks until the ice has melted. Dry the spankee's buttocks if so desired and administer a good spanking to the spankee.

b) After the first spanking is completed, start over with more ice and repeat this until you're done.

IF-THEN – This scenario can be used with adults, particularly in Domestic Discipline relationships. The number of spankings, spanking duration, intensity, length, implement used and number of spankings the spankee gets are set up ahead of time for a wide range of infractions. Over spending on a credit card would have a clear and previously defined punishment, as would being late for work etc. Couples can spend a lot of quality horny-time determining what punishments the submissive member of the relationship would get for which infraction.

IMPULSE SPANKING – Unexpectedly administering a spanking without warning and perhaps for no particular reason.

INSUFFICIENT DISCIPLINE – When the submissive party thinks (to him/herself, or out-loud) that the dominant is not disciplining him/her adequately or is strong enough emotionally to administrate the discipline.

JUICY BUTT – A bottom that likely is great for spanking (or one that someone thinks would be great for spanking.)

KNEADING (aka *Petrissage*) - The palms of the hands and/or fingers work the buttock's muscle and fat tissue. Kneading a spankee's bare buttocks is also popular before, during, and/or after a spanking.

KNICKERS DOWN – An English saying meaning "panties down" in preparation for the spanking she so desperately needs.

LEATHER BUTT - A slang term for buttocks that are comparatively insensitive to spanking and do not mark easily. With enough spankings many buttocks become less sensitive.

LESBIAN SPANKING – When women play with each other sexually, and that includes spanking.

LESBIAN SPANKING STORIES – Erotic girl-girl spanking literature.

LIMIT – The point where the submissive party is unwilling to accept any spanking related additional intensity, duration and/or experience.

LINGERIE SPANKING – Spanking while the pretty lady is wearing lingerie.

KISS OF THE PADDLE – When a blow from a paddle on the butt leaves a significant mark.

LAP-WRIGGLING SPANKING – (a.k.a. *Good Old-fashion Lap-wriggling Spanking*) – Wiggling while over a lap getting spanked. (This is more of an English term.) This wiggling likely is because the spanking is particularly intense or the spankee's ability to take a spanking is not too developed.

LIGHT SPANKING – This can be applied to a clothed or bare bottom. It can be administered by hand or via the use of a spanking implement. It should not be particularly painful for most spankees.

LONG, HARD SPANKING – A lengthy and intense punishment spanking meant to change unacceptable behavior.

MAINTENANCE SPANKINGS – (*Preventative Maintenance Spankings*) - Spankings administered on a regular basis to keep the spankee on the straight and narrow. Punishment spankings are administered in addition to these.

MARATHON SPANKING – Lengthy spanking sessions that might be part of spanking contest or simply for a couple to establish their own personal best. In some marathon spanking sessions the couple can take a short break periodically.

MARKS – (*Spanking Marks*) – A good spanking with more than moderate intensity (depending on how sensitive the spankee's bottom is) can leave the bottom a lovely shade of red. It also can leave light contusions and more significant bruises. These bruises (aka "marks") could remain for days or longer or they can be gone in hours. A spankophile is proud of these marks hence the phrase "wears her (his) marks with pride".

MEMORY RECOVERY SPANKING – Spankings administered to hopefully help the spankee remember things he/she had forgotten. The hope is that he/she can remember that forgotten thing while being spanked or afterwards.

M/f SPANKING – Male spanking female.

MODERATE INTENSITY SPANKING – A spanking administered with only moderate intensyuhui oity typically will give the bottom some or more redness. It shouldn't make the spankee cry or leave marks. This all depends on how sensitive the spankee's ass cheeks are.

MOOD CORRECTION SPANKING – When a spanking(s) is administer to alter the mood of the spankee. Perhaps the spankee is in a bad mood. A mood correction spanking is then administered in an attempt to alter his/her perspective/attitude. More than one mood correction spanking can be given and given between relatively short time intervals.

MOTIVATIONAL SPANKING – This type of spanking scenario can help the spankee reach their goals. Perhaps the goal is good grades in college, or weight loss, or quitting smoking. Motivational spankings can work (but like anything in life is not guaranteed to work.)

(1) Before the spankee embarks on their endeavor he/she can be given the first motivational spanking, which is a serious spanking that really show him/her that it's better to stick with the program. His/her subconscious mind needs to be motivated also and a really good spanking might do just that.

(2) Should the spankee fail to reach previously established goals, he/she should be very soundly spanked and otherwise punished. Other punishments can include corner time, not being allowed to wear cloths (when in private,) Bed Arrest, orgasm denial and other forms of humiliation can also be incorporated. Perhaps you'd also like to invite all your BDSM/kinky friends over to give him/her a spanking.

MUSICAL SPANKING – Spanking to the beat of the music and/or for the length of the musical composition. (Ever spanked to "Bolero"?)

Another great thing about music is that it might cover up the sound of the spanks hitting the spankee's bottom and noises the spankee utters as his/her bottom is reddened.

NAKED SPANKING – The spankee, and optionally the Spanker, are not wearing any cloths.

NSA SPANKING – (No Strings Attached Spanking) – Casual spanking where a special relationship is not necessary.

OLD FASHIONED BARE BOTTOM SPANKING – These are the standard spankings we grew up with. *Silent Spankings* and many if not all spankings when the Spanker is tied down to spanking furniture, likely are not in this category. This term denotes a hard or harder than normal spanking.

OTK – (a.k.a. *OTK Spanking*) – Short for *Over The Knee*. This is one of the most popular spanking positions. Its benefits include that the spanking can start quickly versus having to tie the spankee up. Also the spankee's private parts and ass, with all its features, are in easy reach for the Spanker's use (assuming the spankee allows that.)

PADDLE – A rigid spanking implement that typically is quite a bit longer than it is wide. The thickness of a paddle can vary. Paddles can increase the intensity of the spanking blows and make spanking a less tiring affair for the Spankers. Paddles are usually made of wood but can be made of other hard materials such as acrylic.

PARTY SPANKING – Spanking that takes place at social gatherings. This includes *Spanking Games* and *Group Spankings*. Party Spanking is not the same as *Spanking Parties*.

PLAYFUL SPANKING – This can be when the spankee gets only light to moderate swats or a limited number of quick swats. Consensual playful spankings might be used to break the tension.

POUTING - To make a facial expression that indicates dissatisfaction; sulking. This might be done by the spankee prior to the spanking or when there is an indication that a spanking will take place in the future.

PRIVATE SPANKING - These spankings are given in an isolated private setting with invited company only.

PREVENTATIVE MAINTENANCE SPANKING – See *Maintenance Spanking*.

PROFESSIONAL SPANKING – When money or material goods are exchanged for one or more spankings. Spankings are given professionally by *Spanking Theraphists, FemDoms, Spanking Demonstrators* and others. It could also be the opposite where it's the spanking model that gets spanked in exchange for money or material goods. (This includes spanking pictures and spanking video models.) *Charity Spanking* is when people are spanked in exchange for others giving money to one or more charities for each good spank the spankee takes.

PUBLIC SPANKING – (This includes *Exhibition Spanking*) – Spankings given in a public or semi public non-group spanking environment. (Not recommended!)

PUNISHMENT AGREEMENT – A *Punishment Agreement* is an oral or written agreement that defines what punishments will be given for what offenses. See *Spanking Contract* and *BDSM Contract*.

PUNISHMENT FETISH – The idea of being punished, or even of being punished in a certain way (such as being spanked) in some way turns on the individual and could be a re-occurring fantasy.

PUNISHMENT ROOM – A room, or area of a room (often the basement, bedroom or the dominant's study) where most of the spankings take place.

PUNISHMENT SPANKING - (*Discipline Spanking*) – These spankings leave the spankee's bottom red and marked. These are hard spankings meant to change a wayward spankee's behavior. Typically the female spankee (and sometimes male) will cry from these. Also applied as part of the punishment could be corntime, bedroom time and other punishments. Perhaps the spankee will only be allowed to crawl for the rest of the day/night if going somewhere in the house, (obviously privacy is required.) Maybe one punishment spanking will not be enough, or even two! The subconscious mind needs to know what he or she did is no longer allowed!

PURIFICATION RITUAL SPANKING – This spanking category is more on the spiritual side. It can combine enemas, massage, prayer, meditation and/or bathing for spiritual arousal and/or renewal.

PUSSY SPANKING – The vagina is lightly spanked for stimulation and/or punishment.

QUICKIE SPANKING – When time is limited, but the spankee must have a spanking, he/she can be bent over the nearest applicable furniture or go over your lap for an immediate spanking. Often this is when the spankee is already dressed for an occasion. A quickie spanking needs to be given instantly, likely without any significant preparation, waiting time, discussion, or scolding.

REAL TEARS – This indicates that what's occurring is a good hard spanking! Sometimes during a spanking video shoot, the spankee, in-between takes, has a bit of water put by her eyes to mimic tears. No need to do that when the tears are real!

RED BOTTOM SPANKING - (a.k.a. *Red Ass Spanking*) – A good spanking should leave the spankee with some or more redness on his/her bottom. A bottom that is covered with redness would be from a true *Red Bottom Spanking* that the spankee can 'wear' with pride! The red bottom may be accompanied with marks (bruises).

RELIGIOUS SPANKING – Religious spanking has a very long history. Men and women's buttocks have been beaten for, and by, religious authorities in many past civilizations. Certain members of Christian clergy are recorded to have spanked (women in particular) back when it was easier for them to get away with it. Inquisitioners would beat men and women, often without mercy, as they considered them to be an affront to god.

A part of religious spanking history that may be of interest is how often women in the medieval and post medieval centuries, (often coupled women,) would request a spanking from the clergy (such as their minister or priest) as atonement for their sins or as confidential punishment for something isolated that they did. Often their husbands okayed it. Heck it was a lot better than going to hell right, at least that was what they thought.

Some church building basements had a separate section for these atonement sessions. This happened more often than people realize.

REWARD SPANKING – (1) When a spankophile just can't get enough spankings that you are actually able to reward her/him by giving a spanking. (2) A FemDom might consider all spankings she gives to her slaves to be a reward, or should be viewed as a reward. Punishment for bad behavior is typically more severe than a reward spanking.

ROMANCE SPANKING - This is for spanking couples involved in a romantic relationship. The spanking can be mixed with sexual stimulation and intercourse.

RULER – (Wooden Ruler) – Though often made of wood, it can be made of other substances. Some rulers are thicker than others and somewhat longer than one foot. The thick 1½ foot ruler is a dandy! The yardstick can be very useful for those long reaches, for instance when the naughty girl is sucking on a man's cock and he wants to spank her at the same time. (Watch out for those teeth!)

SAFE SPANKING – Don't spank too hard. Some spankees' butts are able to take more abuse than others, at least until the butt toughens up (assuming it does.) Also you want all parties to feel secure with the location and privacy of the place selected for the spanking.

SANDPAPER CHAIR – After the spankee is spanked, he or she sits naked on sandpaper. An alternative is to rub sandpaper on the spankee's well spanked bottom and/or run your fingernails over the spanked buttocks.

SCHOOLGIRL SPANKING – The naughty (adult) schoolgirl discipline fantasy is one of the most popular spanking fantasies. She is dressed in the pelted skirt and white dress shirt (perhaps also with a tie) and is constantly getting in trouble so she is constantly spanked! All female spanking enthusiasts (spankees) should have a schoolgirl outfit!

SELF-SPANKING – Spanking yourself.

SEXUAL DOMINATION – (Associated with *Sensual Domination*) - The dominant person controls and orchestrates the sexual relationship and sexual activity with the submissive person.

SERIOUS SPANKING – (1) Spanking enthusiasts that take the art of spanking seriously. (2) A hard or even severe spanking and typically is reserved for punishment.

SERVANT SPANKING – (Also see *Slave Spanking*) - Spanking of servants (though in past centuries and millennia they more often were slaves) occurred often. In those days masters and mistresses lorded over their servants with more power than they do today. If the lord (or mistress) of the house thought beating the servant would make good discipline (or simply enjoyed it), that was the servant's fate should she wish to continue working there, or often anywhere else as employment references were important.

The servant girl might be spanked for pleasure by the master of the house. She might be enjoyed in other ways too, though not as often from vaginal intercourse. Servant girls that ended up taking the role of concubines might be treated better and have less mundane work to do. Wives in those days were frigid move often than now. This might be because they were afraid to have too much sex with their husbands as it was so much easier to get pregnant back then thanks largely to a pronounced lack of birth control and the stricter demands of the prevailing religious forces that were staunchly against birth control. (Also women died during childbirth a lot more frequently back then.) A surprising number of wives simply considered the sex demands of their husbands to be too much and welcomed their use of a servant in that manner if it freed them from that arduous duty, (assuming he did not get her pregnant and kept his distance from her emotionally.)

The mistress of the house might order someone to be spanked (beaten) and perhaps do it herself. Husbands and male friends (or other servants) often were happy to do the beating for her, assuming it was a female getting spanked.

The person being beaten may or may not have the area being beaten, fully exposed (thus naked.)

SEVERE SPANKING - This type of spanking can cause much redness and/or severe bruising (marking), blistering or worse on the buttocks of most spankees. The spankee likely will find sitting a challenge for a certain amount of time. This needs to be done in a consensual manner and might not be legal.

SEXUALLY ORIENTED SPANKINGS - Sexually Oriented Spankings are spankings that are specifically given to make the spankee orgasm or at least get as much sexual pleasure as possible.

SILENT SPANKING – (1) When the spankee is not allowed to utter any noise while being spanked. (2) Alternatives to spanking that quietly give the butt pain, such as the application of capsicum cream (but a very small amount) and the less effective Tiger Balm. Do not put it on the anus or sex organs.

SLAVE SPANKING – See *Servant Spanking*. (1) In the modern world of BDSM (*Bondage, Domination, Sadism and Masochism*) the submissive person is called a slave and is under the influence and/or control of the dominate party typically called the "Master" (if male) or "Mistress" if female. The submissive slave is dominated and spanked when the dominant feels it is necessary for discipline and/or pleasure. (2) (See *Servant Spanking* for more on this part of the definition.) Slaves in ancient times often were considered part of the family. They may have been expressly gotten for purposes of physical and sexual pleasure. They were spanked publically and privately in Roman and Greek locations at the whim of their owners. In the more modern slave ownership period including the Caribbean and in North America, black slave girls would also be used for sexual gratification when their owners wanted it. Also other male slaves might spank other slaves for various reasons, particularly when they were a supervisor.

SLIPPERING - Using a slipper as the spanking implement.

SOOTHING CREAM – (Cold Cream) - A cream applied to a well spanked bottom to limit the sensation of pain.

SOUND SPANKING – See *Hard Spanking*.

SPANKABLE – (Spankworthy) – The person is well suited to be spanked. They may appear to have an ass, due to its shape and/or appearance, that appears particularly well designed to be spanked. The mannerisms of the person should scream "spank me"! A professional spanking actress should have great "spankability".

SPANKED TO TEARS – When the spankee is spanked hard enough to cry real tears. Bad girl!

SPANKFEST – A synonym for "Spank Feast". This is a gathering, public or private, where spanking is one of the primary events (or at least is publicized to be.)

SPANKING ART - (Spanking Comics) – Spanking themed art.

SPANKING AGREEMENT - An oral or written agreement regarding spanking related activities. See *Spanking Contracts*.

SPANKING BEGINNERS – *Spanking Beginners* typically have little or no significant experience with giving a spanking and/or receiving a spanking.

It's important that the beginner's first spanking (or first few spankings) are as positive an experience as possible. Does the spankee want it to be a sexual experience also, if so then make sure sexual stimulation is accented. A bad experience now could turn this person off from spanking and another butt is lost to the spanking world :(

SPANKING BLOG – A (preferably) regularly updated online diary/web magazine that individuals and organizations keep regarding spanking pursuits.

SPANKING BONDAGE - When bondage is included with the spanking. Typically this means that the spankee is securely tied down and immobile for his/her spanking. Perhaps he/she is tied down to a piece of spanking furniture.

SPANKING CLUB – These associations provide a way to meet and/or otherwise intertwine with others in the spanking scene. They're sometimes called "Munches". Spanking clubs have grown quite a bit in number in recent years.

SPANKING CONTEST – When couples compete with spankings for a prize or prizes. The rules vary from contest to contest. Possibly included are:

A) Extra points for the spankee with the reddest butt
B) Extra points for the nicest looking marks
C) Points deducted for blistering or appearance of blood (typically then the spanking is over for them anyway)
D) Extra points for sexiest spankee's behavior while being spanked.
E) Points deducted for the spankee trying to block blows or get away
F) Points deducted for the Spanker tiring too quickly
G) Extra points for the spankee with the sexist outfit and/or the outfit most conducive to making the spanking easier
H) Extra points for the Spanker/spankee couple that is the most fun to listen to during the spanking
I) Extra points for how sexy and submissive the spankee is during and at the end of the spanking. She will have to beg for forgiveness, etc.
J) Extra points to the couple that uses the most spanking implements during the spanking
K) Extra points to the spankee's bottom that feels the best after being well spanked.
L) Extra points to the spankee that gets the most aroused
M) Extra points for the spankee with the most spanks during that time period.

Multiple spankings can be going on at the same time. Also see *Duel Spanking*.

SPANKING CONTRACT - It's a good idea for the participants to sit down and talk about their spanking scenarios, including under what circumstances the spanking will take place, how the spanking will be delivered, number of swats, instruments to be used, position of the person to be spanked, whether spanked with clothing on or bare bottom, etc. All participants then have an oral agreement on the terms, or have a signed written contract on the terms. This author sells a *Spanking Contract* through your ebookstore.

SPANKING CURRENCY - This is when spanks take the place of money, more specifically in place of your country's currency. How many spanks do you have in your spanking account? What are you going to buy with them? Or perhaps you are making a trade? Do you have a debt to pay off?

A common "spanking currency" scenario is paying off a debt. The spankee gets spanked in exchange for the debt.

SPANKING DANCE –The sub/slave does a sexy dance in front of her dominant and is spanked at various parts (times) of her dance. Perhaps it's after the end of each song, or if her dancing is not of an acceptable nature.

SPANKING DEMONSTRATION - When spanking partners demonstrate various aspects of spanking, including spanking implements and the best ways to spank.

SPANKING ENTHUSIAST – (Spankophile) - Someone who enjoys spanking, either receiving or giving. This includes activities related to spanking such as spanking media, building spanking furniture and spanking modeling.

SPANKING FANTASY – (Spanking Fantasies) – Mental images that run through one's head associated with spanking. A great many people have these.

SPANKING FOR COUPLES – Adult spanking activities that couples involve themselves in.

SPANKING FURNITURE – These apparatuses are used to place and secure one or more spankees. These include whipping benches, the spanking horse, the birching horse and the spanking bench. The spankee may or may not be tied down to it. The spankee often will find him or herself in the kneeling position or bent-over position. There should be easy access to their buttocks and often spanking furniture make the buttocks the most elevated portion of the spankee's body. Also being able to take and/or play with the spankee sexually while on and/or tied to spanking furniture is of pronounced importance.

SPANKING GAMES – (1) Online interactive games where the players determine who gets spanked and the intensity of the spankings. A spanking game may let the player interactively spank one or more characters. (2) Physical games such as Strip Poker that calls for one or more participants being spanked at various intervals. This type of spanking game typically has a way of determining who the spankee is and who the Spanker is.

SPANKING HOST – The host or hostess at spanking social events and online and real-life spanking clubs.

SPANKING IMPLEMENTS – These physical devices are used to aid and enhance the delivery of the spanking blows. Examples include paddles, straps, slappers, floggers, rods, switches, canes, spanksticks, crops, the tawse and whips. Not everybody agrees but some people feel this category also includes restraint aids such as handcuffs and rope.

SPANKING LIFESTYLE – The world of spanking is innately intertwined into the lives of the Spanker and/or spankee.

SPANKING MAGAZINE – Content from these wonderful periodicals now are often also online.

SPANKING MASSAGES – Combining full or partial body massages with spankings. The massaging may be the primary activity or vice versa.

SPANKING MASTURBATION – (1) Masturbating during and/or after a spanking and masturbating on those days afterwards while your bottom is still sore from the spanking. (2) Being spanked for masturbating.

SPANKING ORGASM – An orgasm that is obtained while one is being spanked, or while their buttock is still smarting from having been spanked in hours or days since the spanking.

SPANKING PARTY – Spanking parties might be in a home, a hotels or resort and are a gatherings specifically set up to accommodate spanking. Often there tends to be a significantly higher percentage of males at these events than females.

SPANKING POSITIONS – The bodily location of Spanker and spankee just prior to, during and just after the spanking.

SPANKING PRACTIONER – See *Spanking Enthusiast.*

SPANKING REMINDER – This often is a short but relatively intense spanking session to make sure the spankee remembers to be obedient and/or is reminded as to what kind of punishment awaits her should she do something wrong.

SPANKING ROLEPLAY - There are many role-play scenarios that can include spanking. Naughty nurse, submissive maid, naughty schoolgirl, misbehaving cheerleader and warden/prisoner role playing is popular with male dominants and female submissives.

Spanking Roleplaying can require acting and props but it always includes a generous helpings of spankings.

SPANKING SERIES – A sequence and/or collection of spankings and/or spanking characters, stories, videos and/or pictures, which have certain characteristics in common.

SPANKING SESSION – Most associated with visits to FemDoms and Spanking Therapists. These are often "visits" that have a purpose but it still can be just a girlfriend and boyfriend meeting for fun.

SPANKING STICK – These look a lot like manmade canes.

SPANKING STORIES – (*Spanking Novels, Spanking Novellas, Spanking Series, Corporal Punishment Fiction, Flagellation Erotica, Romantic Spanking Stories*) – These are literature adventures involving spanking. These go back to the 1700s and may or may not involve sexual activities. The Marquis de Sade is among the most famous of these authors. In the past these tended to be clandestine publications that were sold secretly.

SPANKING THERAPIST – A person that administers *Spanking Therapy.*

SPANKING THERAPY – This aims to help spankees improve themselves. Perhaps he/she needs more motivation or just the tension release of a good spanking. The spanking is conducted by a professional. The spankee's needs are assessed and addressed in a controlled, nurturing environment (assuming nurturing is what the spankee wants.)

SPANKING VIDEOS – Spanking videos have proliferated with the Internet. As is obvious, these videos show spankees getting spanked and often dominated in other ways.

SPANKING WITH **ANAL STIMULATION** – (1) Directly stimulating the anus while giving a spanking (which can include aiming the blows at the anus and/or to make the blows include the anus.) It can occur before a spanking, and/or in between spankings, and/or after a spanking. This might involve inserting a butt plug (inflatable or otherwise), finger(s), anal vibrator, a dildo, or rectal thermometer into the anus. It might include carefully spanking a dildo that's already put into the anus to make it move up and down in the anus as blows are applied to it and the buttocks. (2) Actually spanking the anus with a narrow spanking instrument. (Spanking related enemas are a separate subject, see *Enema Spanking.*)

Anal stimulation doesn't necessarily include anal intercourse.

SPANKING THE MONKEY – Male masturbation.

SPANKOPHILE – – (*aka Spanking Enthusiast*) - Someone who enjoys spanking, either receiving or giving. Their interest could also include spanking implements, discussing spanking, spanking media, building spanking furniture and spanking modeling.

SPENCER SPANKING PLAN – A well known domestic discipline spanking contract that originated in the 1930s.

STING AND THUD - Thinner spanking instruments such as switches release their energy closer to the skin and thus 'sting' more. Thicker spanking instruments such as paddles release their energy down further in the buttocks making more of a "thud" sensation.

STRAP – (aka *Leather Strap*) – A spanking instrument of various sizes that can be deliciously effective. It's often made of leather and thus is pliable.

STRESS RELIEF SPANKING – (*Tension Relief Spanking*) - The aim of these spankings are to eliminate frustration and guilt and cleanse oneself mentally. At the conclusion of these spankings relaxation and comfort can be had by the spankee.

STRUGGLING – When the spankee fails to hold his/herself adequately in place for/during and after their spanking.

SUBMISSIVE SPANKING – When the spankee wants to feel dominated as part of the spanking, over and above the domination involved with him/her getting spanked.

SUBMIT AND OBEY – A Dom/sub lifestyle outlook where the submissive submits and obeys his/her Dominant.

SWITCH SPANKING – Where the Spanker and spankee take turns spanking each other.

SWITCHING – (Associated with Birching) – A switch is a flexible thin branch (rod) from one or more trees. (A collection of thin branches can be tied together to also be used as a spanking implement.) A switch is applied with force to the buttocks of the spankee. The switch like the cane can hurt more than many other spanking implements due to its thinner surface area so caution is advised. Also see *Caning*.

TENDER – The tendency for the buttocks to become sensitive to the touch after a good spanking.

TENSION RELIEF SPANKING – See *Stress Relief Spanking*.

THRASHING – This term is more popular in England and denotes a hard spanking/beating often with one or more implements.

TICKLE SPANKING – (1) Tickling the buttocks and then spanking it (an act that can be repeated.) (2) Tickling various parts of a person's body such as their belly and the bottoms of their feet, and also spanking that person's buttocks, alternatively or simultaneously.

TIT WHIPPING – Spanking the breasts of a woman using one or more implements. This can only be done consensually and with caution.

TRADITIONAL SPANKING – This denotes standard methods of spanking. No unusual methods of buttocal pain infliction, such as *Silent Spanking*, would be included in this category.

TOP UP SPANKING – These are given regularly, even every few days, even in addition to any other spankings the spankee has received. These spankings are for bad behavior that the spankee got away with during that time period (say week) and for bad behavior she might be tempted to do in the following week. See *Maintenance Spanking*.

TOUCH-YOUR-TOES – When in a standing position the spankee may be ordered to reach down and touch as close to their toes (perhaps their knees) as possible so their buttocks can tighten and stick out thus becoming an easier target to spank.

TOUGHEN-UP SPANKING – These spankings (and spankings in general) if given with regularity, can dull nerve endings in the buttocks as well as toughen tissues in the buttocks. The spankee might evolve into having a "leather butt" which is a butt that can take a disproportionately hard spanking.

WAKE-UP SPANKING – This well helps to wake up sleepy beauty and typically works much better than an alarm clock.

WARM-UP SPANKING - This is a light spanking, often by hand and perhaps on a clothed bottom, before the "real" and more intense spanking begins. Its purpose is to prepare the butt for the coming onslaught.

WEARS HER (HIS) MARKS WITH PRIDE – (*Spanking Marks*) – A good spanking with more than moderate intensity (depending on how sensitive the spankee's bottom is) can leave the bottom a lovely shade of red. It also can leave light contusions and more significant bruises. These bruises (aka "marks") could remain for days or longer or they can be gone in hours. A spankophile is proud of these marks hence the phrase "wears her (his) marks with pride".

WEIGHT-LOSS SPANKING – If the spankee needs motivation to lose weight, spanking can be of use. The spankee can be spanked whenever weight loss goals are not reached and/or can have the more desirable reward of a pleasurable spanking when the goals are met. Perhaps the spankee should be given a hard spanking just before the diet is to begin to remind him/her what's in store if transgressions occur.

WELL-SPANKED BUTT – A buttocks that has the tell-tale signs of having gotten a good spanking.

WET SPANKING – For this the spankee's butt is made wet. It can also be when the spankee wears something wet that covers her bottom and is spanked over that. This can enhance the pain coefficient.

WHEEL BARROW SPANKING POSITION – The Spanker sits up and the spankee lays her hands on the floor directly in front of the Spanker. The spankee spreads her legs and brings her ass and legs up over the sitting Spanker's lap. Her legs are positioned on each side of his upper torso. Her pussy and anus are spread wide open next to his midsection. Her ass cheeks are on his lap, her spread open pussy lips are facing him.

WHEEL BARROW SPANKING – When the entire spanking is administered with the spankee in the wheel barrow spanking position (see previous definition.)

WHUPPIN – Slang for whipping.

WOODEN SPOON – This kitchen implement can also double as a spanking implement. Bad girl!

End

Bed Arrest, the Punishment For BDSM Enthusiasts

By Phil G.

Copyright (C) 2013

Book #3

Defining Bed Arrest

Thank you for reading this book, the first book on bed arrest.

This punishment technique can only be used when all parties involved have fully consented to it.

For consistency's sake, this book discusses bed arrest where the punisher is a male master and the person being sentenced to bed arrest is a female submissive or slave. Bed arrest as a punishment can however work just as well in situations when the two parties involved are of the same sex.

I am honored to say that as a master I have incorporated bed arrest into my relationships many times. I have found that it can be a useful tool for changing errant sub/slave behavior.

In this book I'll also make suggestions regarding how (in my opinion) to most optimally carry out the sentence of bed arrest on a sub/slave. Obviously both parties involved can adapt what's in this book to fit their desires, needs and time schedule.

This book also assumes (for all involved) that the sub/slave will accept being put in bed arrest and obey her master's rules associated with it. Obviously if master tells his sub/slave she's just been sentenced to 10 hours house arrest and she points at him and laughs, then master has a problem.

General Definition - Bed arrest is when a master in a BDSM (or related) relationship orders (thus requires) his sub/slave to stay on her bed at all times other than emergencies, and for those additional activities specified. During the time that she is reprimanded to the bed, master may also punish her in other ways such as spanking. He can also play with her, and of course enjoy her sexually.

Bed arrest, as is obvious, is a lot like an adult version of timeout. It doesn't need to be for a longtime; a 30 minute bed arrest session might get the point across just as well. Still all bed arrests sessions are not the same and the sub's restrictions during her incarceration can make all the difference in the world. However beware guys, with her helplessly stuck there, will you be able to resist playing with her all afternoon? (Let's hope she doesn't consider that punishment.)

During bed arrest her freedom can be seriously restricted and she will have time to think about the importance of changing her errant ways.

I gave many 2 day sentences as well as 30 minute sentences. The longest bed arrest sentence I ever given a sub/slave was 4 days. On many occasions I commuted the sentence down because of good behavior, and/or something unexpected came up and/or her sexy begging finally got to me.

Bed arrest in and of itself might not be considered that extreme a punishment. The liberties that the sub/slave loses during bed arrest as well as other punishments she might also experience during that time perhaps can better determine how well she learns her lesson.

1. When to use bed arrest as a punishment. Perhaps your lovely lady has not been reacting well enough to your usual punishments. Perhaps spanking her used to work well as a punishment but now she gets so turned on by it that if anything she'll misbehave to get a good spanking. Finding a new punishment thus has become a necessity.

2. Length of time for putting the sub/slave in bed arrest. Obviously this varies by what extent she needs to be punished and what her and her master's obligations in life are during that time. (Does she have to go to work? Does she have college classes, etc.?)

As she will be allowed out of the bed (and home) for work and other responsibilities, likely that would mean an increase in the length of her sentence as she would be spending less time in bed arrest overall than a sub/slave that could stay around the home all or most of the day.

My experience (and yours may be quite different) is that if the sub/slave has never served a bed arrest, she may have fantasies associated with it.

3. What the sub/slave is allowed to do during bed arrest – How strict and restrictive will her sentence be, at least for the first half or so? Will she need permission to leave the bed for any reason (with the obvious exception of emergencies) including going to the bathroom?

The general rule of thumb is that the less you allow her to do during bed arrest, the more effective the punishment. During the sentence master can progressively give her back more privileges, such as no longer needing permission to go to the bathroom, watch TV, play videogames, watch movies, read books, use the phone, etc. Also was she tied to the bed at all times? Maybe now she can be unbound. (I would strongly suggest that except for emergencies she is never allowed to use the phone during bed arrest.)

My experience is that it's best to start the bed arrest with her having as few privileges as possible and being bound securely to the bed. You then give privileges back as she earns them and/or begs enough for them.

As it's likely you will let her out of the bed to fix meals and do other chores, you'll then need to make sure she's not taking unusually long to do those activities. If so master may want to threaten her with extending her sentence or perhaps another good spanking will take care of that problem.

4. Bondage and blindfolding during her incarceration. Will she be tied up and/or tied to the bed in bondage for a significant amount of the sentence? I would suggest she is and for a substantial amount of time, at least in the first half or more of her incarceration. Blindfolds can help make her feel more isolated and increase the impact of the punishment. Master will probably want to tie her hands in manner so that she **can't** take the blindfold off when she thinks master is not looking, or at least lower the blindfold a bit to look around real quick. Obviously a respectful, well trained sub/slave should not do this but sub/slaves are after all human.

5) Sub/slave needing permission from her master to leave the bed for anything (other than emergencies.) It may seem harsh but my experience is that bed arrest as a punishment works best when to leave the bed for even essential activities, such as going to the bathroom, the sub/slave first needs to have permission from her master. Because of this the master will find that he will need to be in the dwelling and at earshot at all times, just incase, which obviously could be inconvenient for him. With good behavior on her part, this restriction can be lessened.

6) Master will always determine what she does or doesn't wear during the period of bed arrest. *(This is of course is subject to how cold it is, if company shows up and/or if she has to go out of the house for work or other essential activities.)*

During bed arrest, while in private, it's suggested that she not be allowed to wear any clothing.

During the period of her incarceration, also perhaps remove her authority to wear panties while she is out of the house/apartment doing essential public activities such as work and shopping. *(Don't be surprised if she won't go along with this, particularly if it entails doing this at work. If that's the case guys, let it go.)*

7) Pouting, sulking and possibly rebelling by the sub/slave. Master should prepare for his sub/slave to possibly pout, sulk, and as a lengthy sentence progresses, maybe even try to rebel, though hopefully without going too far. Of course the more time master spends with her in bed, playing with her, spanking her, taking her being massaged by her, lying in bed with her, the happier she'll likely be but perhaps the punishment will be less effective, (or perhaps it could have just the opposite effect and be of good benefit).

It's possible that she will rebel to the point that she says she hates you and leaves the house frustrated. It is her right guys and you can't stop her, unfortunately it's likely also a sign of problems in the relationship, and/or a poorly trained sub/slave and/or a sub/slave that simply does not allow herself to be punished with bed arrest, (and/or perhaps other punishments you include during bed arrest.)

Still perhaps she has had a bad experience with bed arrest in the past? That will have to be dealt with in a responsible, respectful manner.

What if she doesn't like bondage and/or blindfolding then either she takes the plunge and lets you do that to her or you don't do those activities.

Perhaps she has obligations that she feels will interfere with the length of her sentence. You would need to let her off for those obligations anyway and perhaps she doesn't understand that.

On the other hand you as master might now find out that she is not a respectful sub/slave, an immature sub/slave and/or too much of a bratty sub/slave and you should find another.

8) Adding more time to her sentence as well as commuting her sentence. The sub/slave should be aware that more time can be added to her sentence. Additionally privileges might not be returned to her as fast during her sentence if she continues to be a bad girl and/or doesn't seem to be learning her lesson.

On the other hand, if she displays a respectful attitude and takes her punishment respectfully then the opposite can occur. Time can be taken off her sentence, and privileges can be returned more quickly during her sentence.

9. How often can we play while she is in bed arrest? Well guys, she's tied up to the bed, naked and blindfolded, good luck keeping your hands off of her! Still the master isn't the one being punished here so his needs and pleasure shouldn't suffer. If he wants his sub/slave to massage him, she should massage him. If he wants fellatio from his sub/slave, by all means get it. If he wants to take his slave, by all means take her. Still it breaks the monotony for her which might not be as conducive to punishment. But it will likely will give her pleasure, make her feel more wanted and loved. Hopefully that won't interfere with her learning her lesson and it might in fact help. Perhaps playing with her later during her incarceration is the better choice, if the master can hold out that long.

Hopefully throughout her sentence she will be on her best behavior in an attempt to get her sentence reduced.

10. What activities can the sub/slave do while she is in bed arrest?

A) Of course her work and parental responsibilities are fully allowed. (If you're living with kids, as you can imagine this punishment could be difficult to perform.)

Still master must watch to make sure she doesn't spend more time than she ordinarily would with her responsibilities. When that's the case her master may wish to add time to her incarceration and/or punish her in other ways.

B) She is required to satisfy her master's sexual desires as always as well as any other activities that can be performed on the bed that she would ordinarily do for her master. This includes massaging her master.

C) Her master perhaps may still also want to punish her in one or more other manners.

11. Privileges that can be taken away from the sub/slave during bed arrest include (depending on circumstances):

*Being able to enjoy video entertainment such as playing video games, watching videos, TV, movies, etc. That can include her favorite programming that would come on during her period of incarceration. (It can be recorded to be watched after her sentence is over.)

*Being able to talk (unless there is an emergency) or she needs permission to do something.

*Being able to use the phone.

*Being able to write things by hand.

*Being able to read for entertainment, such as books.

*Being allowed to have orgasms or otherwise pleasure herself (but dude that's harsh!)

12. Do you close the door on her during her confinement?
No, but it's the master's choice if she's allowed to look at him.

13. How to react to her begging during incarceration. If your sub/slave is adept at begging and if they can be real sexy while doing it, masters may have to ban begging during bed arrest altogether or deal with the horniness that comes with it.

I for one like it when she begs and you can require a certain number of "begs" from her before you'll even consider commuting her sentence.

14. Additional punishments while she is in bed arrest. Perhaps you would like to give her "hourlies". These are spankings given every hour during a set period. She needs to make sure that her master knows it is time for her hourly spanking (or other prescribed hourly punishment) or risk having addition time added to her sentence.

15. Additional general advice to the master. Guys you need to hold strong and be firm. That can be tough. Make sure she takes you seriously throughout this period.

The End